PERCEPTUAL-MOTOR DEVELOPMENT GUIDE

by

MELINDA BOSSENMEYER

EDITOR
Frank Alexander

ARTIST
Dawn Bates

Published by FRONT ROW EXPERIENCE, 540 Discovery Bay Blvd., Byron, CA 94514

1300 BOOKS IN PRINT AS OF 1988

ISBN 0-915256-24-X

Published

by

FRONT ROW EXPERIENCE
540 Discovery Bay Blvd.
Byron, CA 94514

IN APPRECIATION

A special thanks to Dr. Diane Ross, a University Professor of Motor Learning who inspired me and taught me the theory behind which most of this book is based. She is a great teacher who gives students the confidence to contribute.

A special thanks to good old mom, Joelda Owens. She too believed and taught me to love children and nurture their sense of self.

And finally, but certainly not least, to my dear friend, Karen Ulmer, who proof read and added valuable insight, recommendations and clarifications during my many modifications and revisions of this book.

ABOUT THE AUTHOR

Melinda Bossenmeyer M.S. is a public school educator. She is the mother of two children. She is the owner and director of Kinder/Kids Gym, a childrens' motor development program in Southern California. Her other credits include:

* Consultant for California State Department of Education

* Teacher Trainer for Elementary School Physical Education

* Extension Instructor for Sacramento State University, Sacramento, California

* Consultant for California State Health Related Fitness

* Masters' Degree in Physical Education

* California Teaching Credentials for Physical Education and Adaptive Physical Education

* Research Grant Recipient

* Teaching experience since 1973

TABLE OF CONTENTS

INTRODUCTION

This book contains the ingredients of a uniquely designed motor development program for preschool and elementary school age children. All activities are part of a sequential development program. Listed below are some of the topics emphasized and designed to enrich a child's movements and perceptions. Although these activities will be emphasized, many other activities will be presented as well.

1) Balance

2) Body and Space Awareness

3) Eye-Foot Coordination

4) Hand-Eye Coordination

5) Jumping and Sequencing

6) Locomotor Movements

7) Social Skill Development

8) Small Motor Coordination

9) Skill Development through Primary Games

10) Total Body Coordination

It is my belief that children must feel good about themselves and have the confidence to contribute in order to perform well. This book, therefore, is based on your making each class a POSITIVE place for children to have fun, learn and be praised again, again and again.

Kids will be having so much fun that you may be asked, "Is there more to it than fun and games?". This book is based on a motor skills development program developed for a public elementary school which received the highest attainable ratings from the California School Improvement Review Team in 1981.

Please Note: Feel free to copy the Chapter Checklists and Award Certificates for your own classroom use. However, you need to get written permission from the publisher to copy any of the written material, other than the Chapter Checklists and Award Certificates mentioned above.

Also note that to easily copy the Chapter Checklists and Awards, simply tear them out of the book along the perforations provided. Once you've made your master copies, they can be reinserted by using clear invisible-type mending tape. Or, since all the pages are perforated, you may want to remove all pages and simply keep them loose-leaf fashion in a folder, ring binder or use one metal ring in a corner. This will allow you or an aide to easily remove pages with specific activities without taking the whole book. If extensive use is contemplated, it is recommended that you plastic laminate each page once they've been removed from the book.

UNDERSTANDING HOW CHILDREN LEARN MOTOR SKILLS

It is widely documented and universally accepted among educators that children's motor skills develop with a wide range of variation in terms of chronological age. We do know however, the sequence of skill development appears to progress in an orderly fashion.

Three developmental patterns have been identified by Dauer and Pangrazi in their book, "Dynamic Physical For Elementary School Children".

1) Development in general proceeds from head to foot (cephalocaudally), that is, coordination and management of body parts occur in the upper body before they are observed in the lower. The child can therefore throw before he can kick.

2) Development occurs from inside to outside (proximodistally). For example, the child can control her arm before she can control her hand. She can therefore reach for objects before she can grasp them.

3) Development proceeds from the general to the specific. Gross motor movements occur before fine motor coordination and refined movement patterns. As the child learns motor skills, nonproductive movement is gradually eliminated.

The Three E's of Movement:

Enrichment and Exposure to a wide range of activities which allow in part, for Exploratory movement opportunities are key factors upon which to build your motor development program.

Chapter 1
BALANCE

OBJECTIVES

1) Each student will stand on one foot 5 seconds.

2) Each student will hop on one foot 5 times.

3) Each Student will walk a balance board forward, backward and sideways.

4) Each student will balance on a balance board 3 seconds.

5) Each student will balance on different parts of their body (that is, Stork Stand).

6) Balance while manipulating objects. (That is, bouncing a ball, or balancing a bean bag on head while walking on a balance beam.)

EQUIPMENT NEEDS

Walking Board, balance boards, blocks, bean bags, coordination ladder, and tin can stilts.

INSTRUCTIONAL TIPS

1) Balance is the basis of all movement, therefore balance skills should be introduced into a movement program early and reinforced frequently.

2) Encourage children to walk slowly across the beam, emphasizing control.

3) Visual fixation on a target straight ahead at eye level is important. Children tend to want to watch their feet. This should be discouraged.

4) All activities should be practiced on the floor before they are tried on a piece of equipment, that is, walk on a piece of tape on the floor prior to walking on a walking board.

5) When working with a sensory delayed child, you may find it of benefit to remove the child's shoes for an enhanced tactile experience.

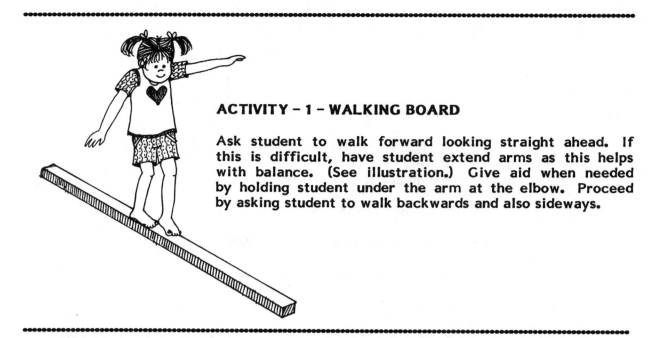

ACTIVITY – 1 – WALKING BOARD

Ask student to walk forward looking straight ahead. If this is difficult, have student extend arms as this helps with balance. (See illustration.) Give aid when needed by holding student under the arm at the elbow. Proceed by asking student to walk backwards and also sideways.

ACTIVITY – 2 – WALKING BOARD

Ask student to verbalize the direction he is walking. Ask him to walk forward to the end and without turning around, to walk backwards back to the beginning. The next step is to ask the child to walk to the center of the beam and then turn around in the center and walk back as well.

ACTIVITY – 3 – WALKING BOARD

Ask the student to walk forward to the center of the beam, bend over and pick up a bean bag and continue walking. Walk the length of the beam, balancing the bean bag on your head or hand.

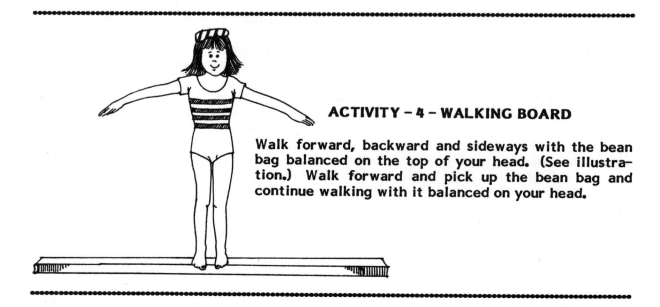

ACTIVITY – 4 – WALKING BOARD

Walk forward, backward and sideways with the bean bag balanced on the top of your head. (See illustration.) Walk forward and pick up the bean bag and continue walking with it balanced on your head.

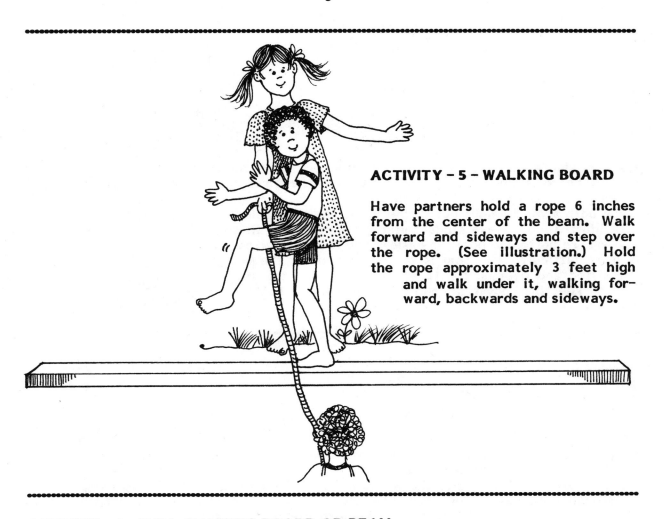

ACTIVITY – 5 – WALKING BOARD

Have partners hold a rope 6 inches from the center of the beam. Walk forward and sideways and step over the rope. (See illustration.) Hold the rope approximately 3 feet high and walk under it, walking forward, backwards and sideways.

ACTIVITY – 6 – TALL WALKING BOARD OR BEAM

Use the above listed progressions, raising the height as the child becomes more comfortable with height and balance.

ACTIVITY – 7 – WALKING BOARD

Walk forward and bounce a ball in hoops as you are walking. (See illustration.) Crawl through a hulahoop placed on a beam by an assistant without touching the sides of the hoop.

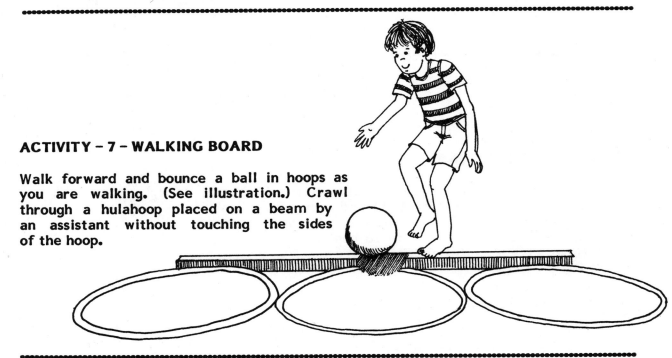

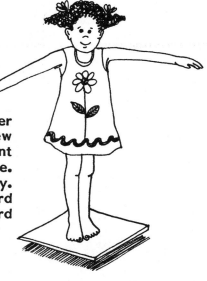

ACTIVITY – 8 – BALANCE BOARDS

Have students get feet as close together in the center of the board as possible. Give assistance the first few times getting onto and off the balance board. Have student place both arms straight out in the air to assist in balance. (See illustration.) Have student step onto the board slowly. The square bottomed board is easiest and the circular board is more difficult. The goal is to get on and off the board unassisted and balance for 10 seconds. Remind the student to keep his body tight and this will assist in balance success.

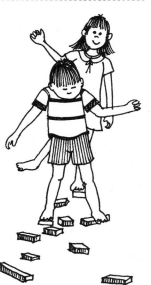

ACTIVITY – 9 – BLOCKS

Scatter blocks in a confined area and ask students to try to successfully "cross the brook" and get to the other side without stepping off the block ("into the water"). (See illustration.) Give all students a chance and then rearrange the formation. This can be made more difficult and to require planning by telling students that they can only step on the red blocks with their right foot and blue blocks with their left foot.

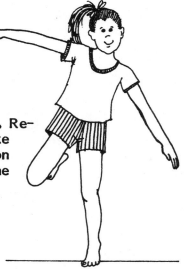

ACTIVITY – 10 – STATIONARY BALANCE

Ask student to stand on one foot and balance for 5 seconds. Remembering to keep their body tight and arms out will make it easier. (See illustration.) Switch and try to balance on the other foot for 5 seconds. Try to hop in one spot on one foot 5 times. Try the other foot.

ACTIVITY – 11 – DYNAMIC BALANCE

Stand on one foot and hop forward one time. Land on that foot and balance for 5 seconds. Do the same with the other foot.

ACTIVITY – 12 – OBJECT BALANCE

Balance the bean bag on the head, sit down, and stand up without dropping the bean bag. Practice walking fast and slow without dropping the bean bag. Practice balancing it on different body parts while moving. (See illustration.)

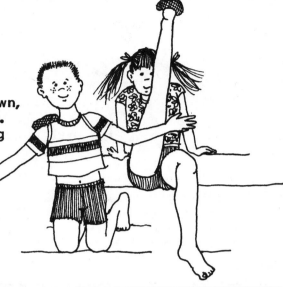

ACTIVITY – 13 – BODY PARTS BALANCE

Place your bean bag on the floor and build a bridge using 4 body parts. Build the bridge high and low. Build a bridge using 2 body parts, etc.

ACTIVITY – 14 – OBJECT BALANCE

Place the bean bag on the instep of your foot. Can you balance the bean bag while swinging your foot forward and backward? (See illustration.) Can you swing your foot up and catch the bean bag with your hand?

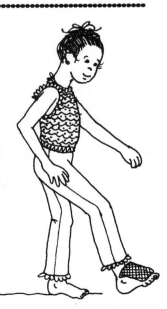

ACTIVITY - 15 - COORDINATION LADDER

The ladder is appropriate for working on many different skills. You will find similar activities listed in other sections. Walk on the rungs of the ladder forward, backwards and sideways.

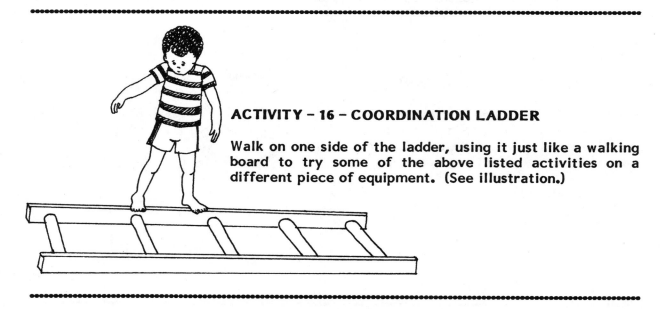

ACTIVITY - 16 - COORDINATION LADDER

Walk on one side of the ladder, using it just like a walking board to try some of the above listed activities on a different piece of equipment. (See illustration.)

ACTIVITY - 17 - COORDINATION LADDER

Creep on hands and feet on the rungs.

ACTIVITY - 18 - BALANCE PUZZLES

Balance puzzles can be made by drawing with a magic marker on the backside of carpet samples. Begin by holding up charts with the various body part symbols and ask children to identify them. Place the balance puzzles in a circle (same number as children in the class). Have each child stand behind a carpet sample and solve his puzzle. After about 10 seconds ask each child to move to the next balance puzzle. Continue until all children have solved each puzzle. (See Balance Puzzle diagram on page 9.)

(Note on page 9 that the "Key" to interpreting the Balance Puzzle is at the top. Also realize that examples of the left hand, right foot, right elbow and left knee were left out of the Key, even though they appear in the puzzle itself. Keep in mind that the basic Key rule is that one color = right and a different color = left with the head and seat having their own distinctive colors.)

- 9 -

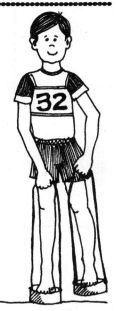

ACTIVITY – 19 – TIN CAN STILTS

Practice first with just one stilt. Practice this way on each foot.
Ask children not to rush or race each other. Practice moving in
different directions and around various obstacles. (See illustration.)

SAFETY FIRST!!

For All Balance Activities Always Be In A Position To Assist Or Spot The Student.

| BALANCE CHECKLIST

NAME	Balance On Right Foot 5 Seconds	Balance On Left Foot 5 Seconds	Walk Balance Beam Forward	Backwards	Sideways	Balance Board 3 Seconds	Stork Stand 3 Seconds	Walking Board Bean Bag On Head	Balance Puzzles				

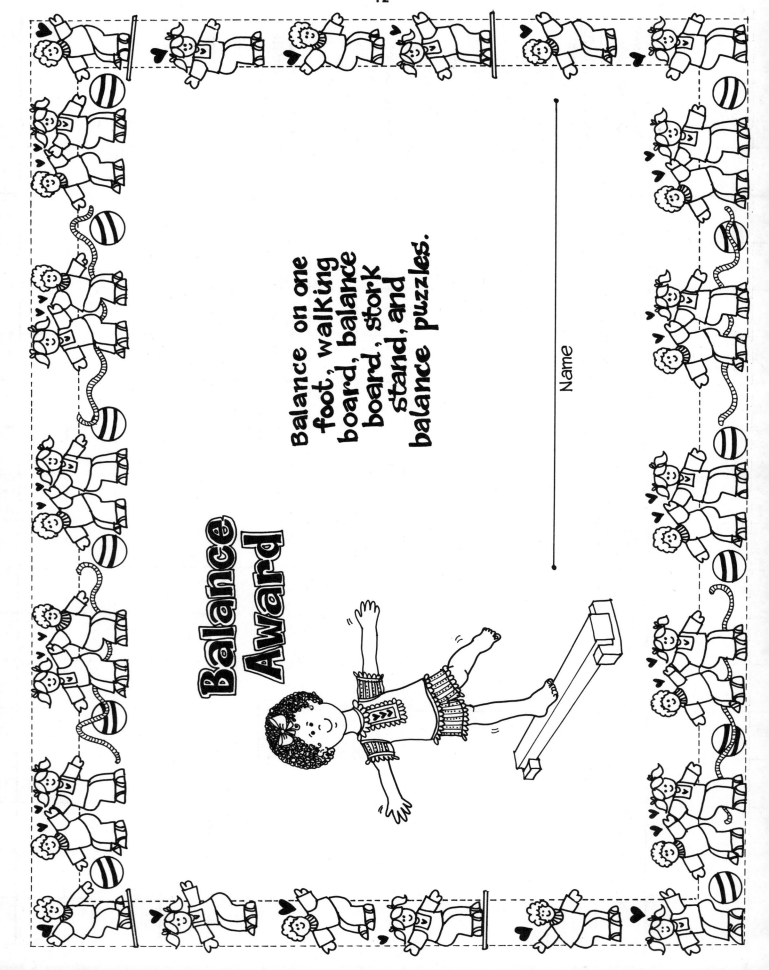

Balance on one
foot, walking
board, balance
board, stork
stand, and
balance puzzles.

Name

Balance
Award

Chapter 2

BODY AND SPACE

OBJECTIVES

1) Each Student will know 10 body parts.

2) Each Student will know 5 parts of the head.

3) Each student will be familiar with directional terms. (That is, in front of, etc.)

4) Students will learn to move their bodies in relation to other objects in the room.

5) Students will follow directional commands while performing locomotor movements.

6) Students will distinguish between left and right.

EQUIPMENT NEEDS

Hoops and geometric shapes.

INSTRUCTIONAL TIPS

1) Children must learn where left and right are in relation to their own bodies before they can learn which is the left and right side of a page (laterality).

2) Children must learn directionality terms in relation to themselves before they can understand relationships of objects in space (external positioning).

●●●

ACTIVITY – 1 – BODY PARTS IDENTIFICATION

Have students close their eyes and identify the following: head, shoulders, knees, toes, elbows, arms, legs, fingers, hands, ankles, wrists, stomach, back, hips, and feet.

●●●

ACTIVITY – 2 – BODY PARTS HEAD

Have students identify the following: eyes, nose, hair, ears, lips, mouth, teeth, eyebrows, chin, cheek, eyelashes, and neck.

●●●

ACTIVITY – 3 – BODY PARTS AND PURPOSES

Have student fill in the blank: My eyes are for_____, My ears are for_____, My mouth is for_____, My feet help me to_____, Etc.

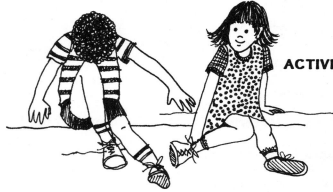

ACTIVITY – 4 – BODY PART TO OTHER BODY PART

Nose to knee, head to shoulder, hand to ankle, knee to knee, fingers to shoulders, wrist to leg, foot to leg, toes to toes, elbow to leg and hand to back. (See illustration.)

ACTIVITY – 5 – DIRECTIONAL TERMS PRACTICE

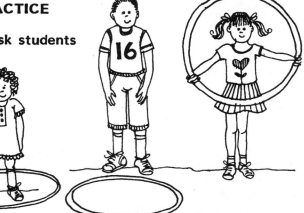

Using hula hoops scattered on the floor, ask students to begin by standing inside their hoop. Continue by presenting the students with the following challenges: Stand in back of the hoop, beside it, hold it over your head, hold it beside you, in front of you, put it on the ground, jump over it. Step inside the hoop, now step outside of the hoop. (See illustration.)

ACTIVITY – 6 – MOVING BODY PARTS IN A SPECIFIC DIRECTION

Have students participate in the following commands: Put your fingers pointing up. Put your head down. Put both arms in front of you. Put one foot in back of you. Put one hand beside you. Put your feet over your head. Put your hands beside your feet. Put your arms in back of your legs. Put your hands besides your ears.

ACTIVITY – 7 – OBSTACLE COURSE ACTIVITIES

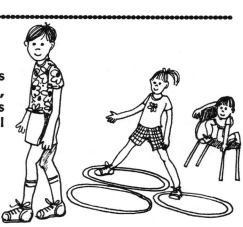

Be creative and invent many different challenges for students by using objects such as chairs, tables, cones, hoops, etc. Body and Space obstacle courses should include something to crawl through, crawl or jump over, something to go under and to go around. Use geometric shapes to crawl through and ask students to verbalize what they are doing (that is, I am crawling through the red triangle). (See illustration.)

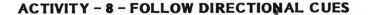

ACTIVITY - 8 - FOLLOW DIRECTIONAL CUES

While performing locomotor movements, ask students to do the following: walk backwards, walk forward, hop forward 4 times, hop backwards, skip forward and then backwards, jump sideways, run forward, run sideways, march forward and walk on your tiptoes backwards.

ACTIVITY - 9 - LATERALITY PRACTICE (LEFT AND RIGHT)

Raise your right hand, left foot, right knee. Touch your right hand to your left knee. Touch your right ear to your right shoulder. Your left foot to your right knee. Walk to the right. To the left. Walk forward and backward.

ACTIVITY - 10 - BODY PARTS GAMES

Play Hokie Pokie, Looby Loo, and Simon Says.

ACTIVITY - 11 - FINGER TALK

I point my finger up. I point my finger down. I point my finger to the front and wave it round and round. Point up, point down, to the back, and round and round. Point up, point down and to the back, and round and round. (Repeat)

ACTIVITY - 12 - BODY PARTS IN ACTION (THE DO IT SONG)

We stamp with our left foot, We stamp with our right, Sing tra la la la la and clap with delight. We look to the left side. We look to the right. Step forward, then backward, and clap with delight.

ACTIVITY - 13 - NUMBER JUMP

I'll jump, 1-2-3. I'll jump, 4-5-6. Now back, 1-2-3. Now up, 4-5-6. I'll jump to the left. I'll jump to the right. I'll jump way up high. Then skip with delight.

ACTIVITY - 14 - HAND SWITCH

This is my right hand. I'll raise it up high, This is my left hand, I'll touch the sky. Right hand, left hand, Roll them around, Left hand, right hand, Pound, pound, pound.

ACTIVITY – 15 – NOBLE DUKE OF YORK

Oh, the noble Duke of York, He had ten thousand men; He marched them up to the top of the hill and marched them down again.

And when you're up, you're up, And when you're down, you're down, And when you're only half way up, You're neither up nor down.

ACTIVITY – 16 – ROCK, BRIDGE, TREE GAME

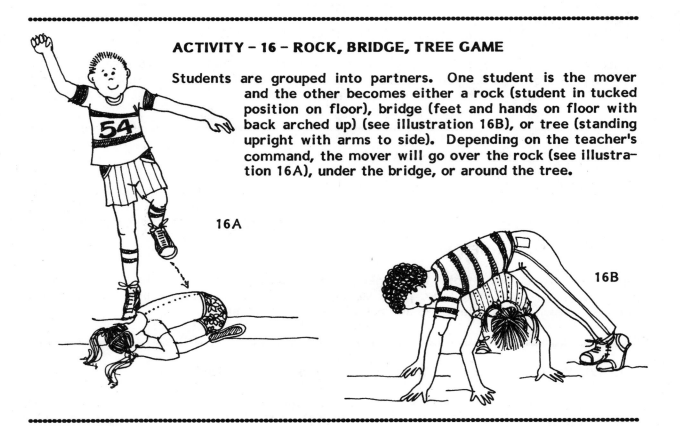

Students are grouped into partners. One student is the mover and the other becomes either a rock (student in tucked position on floor), bridge (feet and hands on floor with back arched up) (see illustration 16B), or tree (standing upright with arms to side). Depending on the teacher's command, the mover will go over the rock (see illustration 16A), under the bridge, or around the tree.

16A

16B

ACTIVITY – 17 – ROCK, BRIDGE, TREE RELAY

Once the concept of over, under and around is clear to the students the class can be divided into small relay teams. Six people for each team will reduce the waiting time. The first person becomes a tree, the second a bridge and the third the rock. The remaining three students become the relay team. On "GO" the first relay person leaps over the rock, goes under the bridge, and around the tree and then back to the end of the line. Once across the end line he must tag the next person. Continue until all children have had a turn.

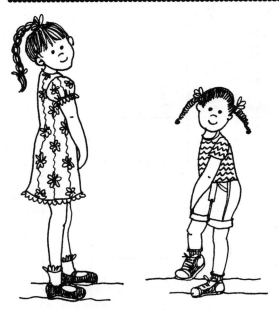

ACTIVITY – 18 – MIRROR IMAGES

Have two students face each other. Ask one student to be the leader and move his arms, or legs slowly so that his partner can easily copy each movement. Continue and let the other partner lead. Switch partners and continue this activity. (See illustration.)

BODY AND SPACE CHECKLIST NAME	10 Body Parts	5 Parts Of Head	Directional Terms Up, Down, Around	Forwards, Backwards, Sideways	Left & Right	In Front Of, Behind	Beside, In, On	Between, Across	Over & Under			

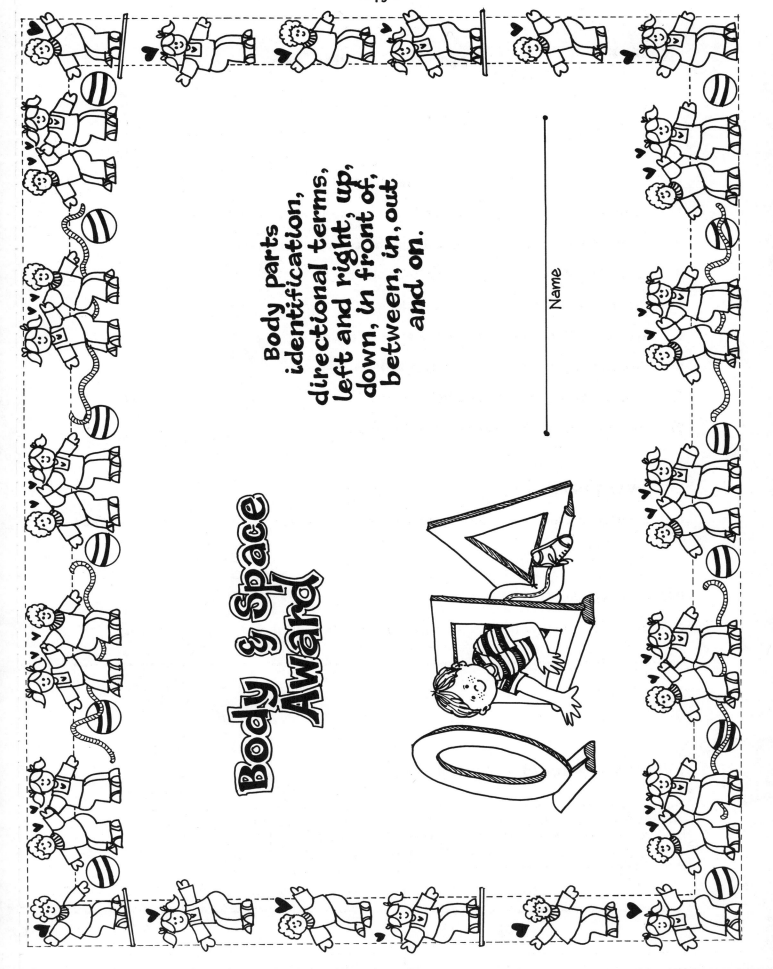

Body & Space
Award

Body parts
identification,
directional terms,
left and right, up,
down, in front of,
between, in, out
and on.

Name

Chapter 3

EYE-FOOT COORDINATION

OBJECTIVES

1) Student will execute a bear crawl on the coordination ladder.

2) Student will execute a rung walk on the coordination ladder.

3) Student will demonstrate hop-scotch skills.

4) Student will demonstrate stilt walking.

5) Student will demonstrate soccer style dribbling.

6) Student will demonstrate jumping skills with a rope.

7) Student will demonstrate block walking.

8) Student will demonstrate kicking for accuracy.

EQUIPMENT NEEDS

Coordination ladder, hoops, stilts, soccer type balls, ropes, balance boards, and bean bags.

INSTRUCTIONAL TIPS

Children often times will not develop a dominate foot until after 5 years of age.

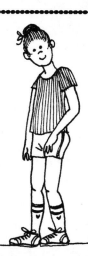

ACTIVITY - 1 - COORDINATION WALKS

Have students find a line on the floor or use a jump rope laid out on the floor for the following activities: 1) Walk forward heel to toe. 2) Walk on your tiptoes. 3) Walk forward with giant steps. 4) Sideways on your tiptoes. and 5) Walk backwards staying on the line or the rope.

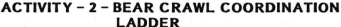

ACTIVITY – 2 – BEAR CRAWL COORDINATION LADDER

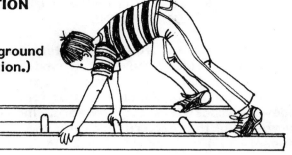

Ask student to practice a bear crawl on the ground by crawling on hands and feet. (See illustration.) Then ask the student to do this same activity on the coordination ladder. The student may then either put his hands on the side of the ladder or the rungs. The side of the ladder is the easiest and should be encouraged first. A more skilled student will be able to go directly to hands and feet on the rungs. Next try hands and feet on the outside supports of the ladder only.

ACTIVITY – 3 – RUNG WALK COORDINATION LADDER

Ask the students to first walk along the side of the ladder like it is a balance beam. Practice walking upright, stepping on the rungs of the ladder. At first, spot each student by holding on under the elbow. As the student becomes more comfortable, ask him to walk sideways and backwards also.

ACTIVITY – 4 – HOPSCOTCH WITH HOOPS

Hopscotch with hoops or with chalk drawn on the blacktop is a good coordination game for children of all ages. If using hoops, ask the students to jump with both feet when there is only one hoop and to spread their feet and jump with one foot in each hoop when there are two hoops side by side. As the students become more skilled, the conventional one foot hop in a single hoop should be encouraged. Use a bean bag and have them perform the same activity only now they throw the bean bag into a hoop and skip it when jumping the pattern. The student who jumps the pattern perfectly gets to pick up his bean bag on the way back and will get another turn.

ACTIVITY – 5 – JUMPING AND SEQUENCING DIRECTIONS

Lay out a tic tac toe like pattern using jump ropes placed on the ground. Ask students to jump the following patterns: forward, forward then sideways or forward, sideways, backwards then forward. Include "across" in the pattern and ask the students to jump the pattern 2 times (3 times, etc.) and then stop.

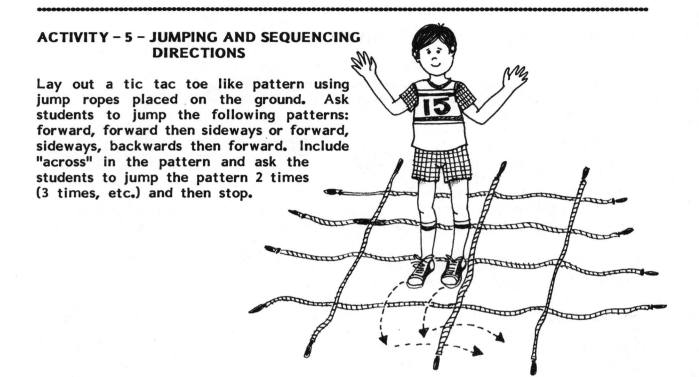

ACTIVITY – 6 – STILT WALKING

Using store-bought stilts or homemade tin can stilts, start by asking the students to walk around with one stilt and get the feel of it. Then progress into practicing with stilts on both feet. Emphasize pulling up with both hands as you walk in order to keep the stilts on.

ACTIVITY – 7 – SOCCER DRIBBLE WITH A NERF BALL

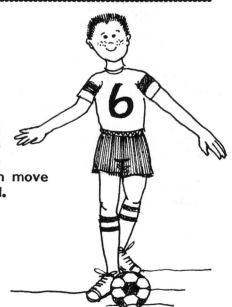

Give each student a nerf ball and show them the correct way to execute a soccer style dribble with the instep of the foot. Have the students dribble around some game cones spaced far apart at the beginning and then move them closer together as the students become more skilled.

ACTIVITY – 8 – JUMPING AND ROPES

All regular jump rope skills require good coordination of the feet. Start by laying a single jump rope out on the ground; one for each child. Ask the students to begin by walking on top of the jump rope. Ask them to then straddle the jump rope and jump on both sides of it. Next have them hop on one foot around the jump rope. When a student can do this rhythmically he is ready for regular jump roping instruction. Stepping across the rope is a good mid-line activity (cross-over walk). Note that it is important to remember that rope jumping is not appropriate until the child is capable of rhythmical jumping on the ground without a rope.

ACTIVITY – 9 – BLOCK WALKING OR OBSTACLE COURSE MOTOR PLANNING

Obstacle courses help with coordination and planning. Regular preschool building blocks work great. Ask students to first walk on the blocks without falling off. You can make this fun by saying, "This is a brook. Don't fall off or you will fall into the water." More difficult patterns require that the child step only on red blocks with his right foot and blue blocks with his left. Obstacle course feet and hand markers are available commercially or can be made. They are also great for motor planning practice.

ACTIVITY – 10 – SOCCER KICK FOR ACCURACY

Set up two game cones and let the students practice kicking a soccer ball through them. Start with the goals wide at the start and then make them more narrow as the child becomes more skilled.

ACTIVITY – 11 – CRAWL THROUGH THE LADDER

Turn the coordination ladder onto its side. Ask student to crawl on hands and knees and go in and out through the rungs of the ladder.

ACTIVITY – 12 – BALANCE BOARDS

Ask students to stand with their arms out and place their feet on the center of the balance board. A spotter should always be placed close to a student on a balance board.

ACTIVITY – 13 – SPACE AWARENESS

Select objects of various heights such as boxes, blocks, etc. Ask the child to step over them without touching them.

ACTIVITY – 14 – BEAN BAG FOOT RELAY

Direct the children to push bean bags across the floor with their feet. Use both feet and pass it on to the next person.

ACTIVITY – 15 – CIRCLE "KEEP IT IN" GAME

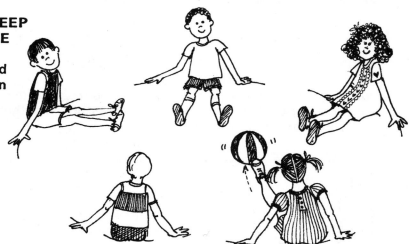

Children sit in a circle and attempt to keep a ball in the circle with their feet. Have the children lean back on their hands with their feet straight ahead. Do not let them touch the ball with their hands.

NAME	Coordination Ladder Bear Crawl	Rung Walk	Hop Scotch (Hoops)	Stilt Walking	Soccer Style Dribbling	Jumping Skills	Block Walking	Kick For Accuracy					

EYE-FOOT CHECKLIST

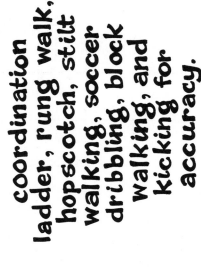

Eye-Foot Award

coordination ladder, rung walk, hopscotch, stilt walking, soccer dribbling, block walking, and kicking for accuracy.

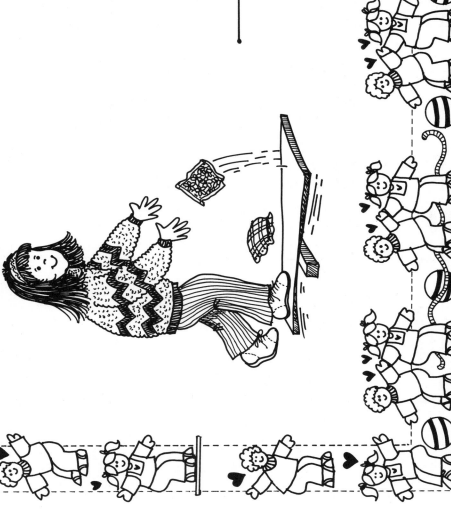

_____
Name

Chapter 4

JUMPING AND SEQUENCING

OBJECTIVES

1) Each student should jump 10 times in one spot.

2) Each student should jump from a jumping box and display correct landing techniques.

3) Each student should be able to jump 10" high.

4) Each student should learn rhythmic jumping without a rope.

5) Each student should be able to jump in various directions following verbal commands.

6) Students 5 years and older should be able to jump a long jump rope.

EQUIPMENT NEEDS

Hoops, jump ropes and jumping box.

INSTRUCTIONAL TIPS

1) Jumping is an excellent activity for coordination and conditioning all parts of the body. It requires good coordination as well as rhythm and timing skills. Rope skipping is a very popular activity for elementary school children. A child is developmentally ready to learn to jump rope around 5 years old.

2) A three year old child is ready to begin jumping skills.

3) Long jump rope skills can be introduced after 5 years old.

4) Most 6 year olds are ready for individual rope jumping.

ACTIVITY - 1 - JUMPING

Ask students to stand inside of a hula hoop and jump up and down 10 times. Can you stay inside the hoop? Can you use the hoop to jump back and forth over the hoop in place? Can you broad jump over your hoop? Jump back and forth around the sides of your hoop all the way around your hoop. Jump getting your feet high off the ground. Now see how low you can keep your feet to the ground and still jump over the side of the hoop. (See illustration.)

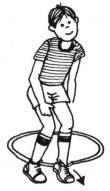 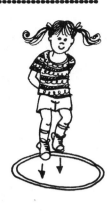

ACTIVITY - 2 - JUMPING ON A ROPE LAID ON THE GROUND

Give each student a rope to lay on the ground. This is an excellent activity for developing balance skills as well as jumping skills. Have students walk forward on the rope heel-toe fashion. Now ask students to straddle the rope and jump forward to the end of the rope. Ask them to hop on one foot around the rope and then switch and hop on the other foot. (See illustration.) Jump forward and backwards over the rope placed on the ground. Jump sideways over the rope with two feet and back again 10 times in place. Repeat, but jump the length of the rope and back again side to side.

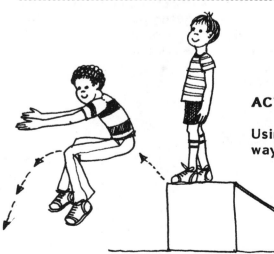

ACTIVITY - 3 - JUMPING BOX

Using a jumping box lets students explore different ways of landing when jumping off the box. Emphasize that letting the knees give and bend makes the landing softer. Arms extended will also help with balance. (See illustration.) Work on sequencing a correct landing followed by a forward roll.

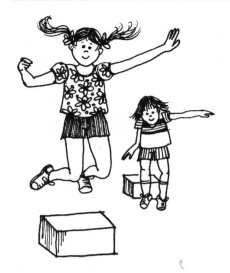

ACTIVITY – 4 – JUMPING OBSTACLE COURSE

Devise an obstacle course where students are required to jump over things, jump across (hoop), jump down from a jumping box (see illustration), broad jump forward and balance on a target, etc.

ACTIVITY – 5 – JUMPING ROPE

Most students at 5 years old can rhythmically jump a long rope that is being turned for them. While the student is actually not "jumping the rope" he will be able to jump it because of learning a rhythmical pattern of jumping. To begin teaching this you tell students that their job is to jump and that your job as a rope turner is to make the rope go under their feet. Ask them to stand in the middle and to begin jumping without the rope being turned. Say "Jump, jump. Jump, jump. Jump, jump.", verbally calling out the pattern for the jumper. When the student is well into the pattern begin turning the rope. Most students are successful with this technique and later, actually through experience learn to jump rope.

ACTIVITY – 6 – JUMPING AND FOLLOWING DIRECTIONS

Play Mother May I and have students request the number of jumps and also the direction they need to travel. Or play Red Light, Green Light. Reinforce the concepts of forward, backward and sideways.

ACTIVITY – 7 – JUMPING WITH A ROPE GRID

Lay ropes out in a tic tac toe pattern on the floor. Ask students to sequence the following commands. Jump forward, forward, across and backwards. Or jump forward, sideways, sideways and forward. Repeat the pattern and let's see where you end up.

JUMPING AND SEQUENCING CHECKLIST NAME	Jump 10 Times	Jump And Land With Absorption	Rhythmic Jumping	Jump Backwards 5 Times	Jump Long Rope 5 yr Olds +	Jump Short Rope 6 yr Olds +	Jump Across Midline 10 Times							

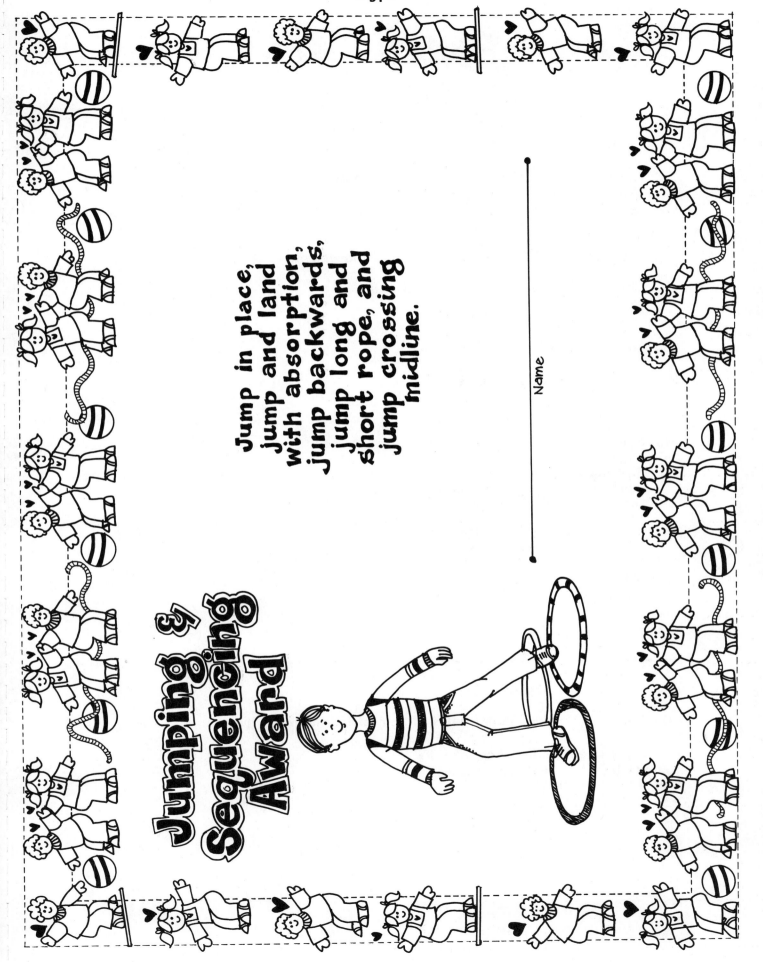

Jumping & Sequencing Award

Jump in place, jump and land with absorption, jump backwards, jump long and short rope, and jump crossing midline.

Name

Chapter 5

LOCOMOTOR SKILLS

OBJECTIVES

1) Each student will learn basic locomotor movements of walk, run, jump and hop.

2) Each student will also learn locomotor movements of skip, gallop and slide.

3) Students will learn various animal walks.

EQUIPMENT NEEDS

Hoops, colored chalk, parachute and music.

INSTRUCTIONAL TIPS

1) Locomotor skills are the foundation of large muscle movements and the cornerstone of gross motor coordination. There are 8 basic locomotor movements which include: walk, run, leap, hop, jump, skip, gallop and slide.

2) When practicing locomotor skills, allow students to rest periodically as they will tire easily with repeated practice.

3) Children should have their head up and eyes forward when practicing a locomotor skill.

••

ACTIVITY – 1 – ANIMAL WALKS

Practice the following animal walks while reciting the following chants:

Big frog, little frog, hop, hop, hop.
Can you be a frog and hop, hop, hop?
(See illustration 1A.)

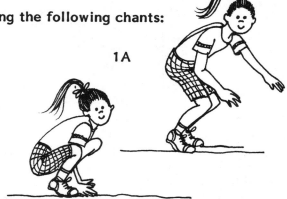

1A

Fe, Fi, Fo, Fair,
Who can be the big brown bear?
(See illustration 1B and see Bear Walk description
on page 34.)

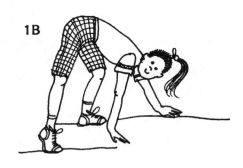

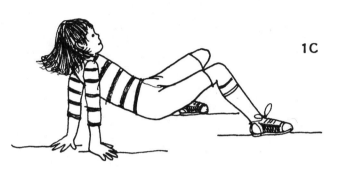

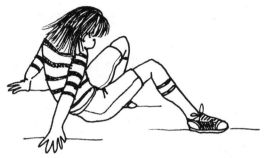

Mr. Crab in the sand.
Up and down he walks around.
(See illustration 1C above and see Crab Walk description on page 34.)

Elephant so big and gray
Can you show how an elephant walks today?
(See illustration 1D at right.)

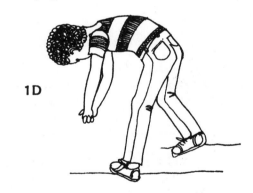

Amy Anteater moves at will,
she lifts one foot
and she stands still.

Closing rhyme:

Have a happy day, you can do it, nothing to it.
Have a happy day all day!

Other animal walks include:

ALLIGATOR CRAWL
Lie face down on the floor with
elbows bent. Move along the
floor alligator fashion keeping the hands close to the body and feet out. (See illustration 1E upper right.)

PUPPY DOG
Walk on all fours with knees and arms bent.

MONKEY RUN
Walk bent at waist with hands turned in. (See illustration 1F at right.)

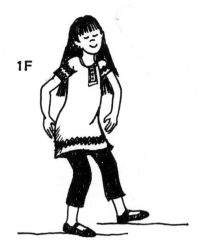

1F

BEAR WALK
Walk on all fours with arms and legs extended. (See previous illustration 1B on page 33.)

INCH WORM
On all fours walk feet up to hands and then walk hands away from feet while keeping feet planted. Then reverse it and keep hands planted while your feet catch up with your hands. (See illustration 1G below.)

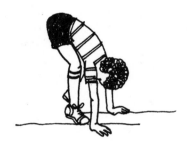 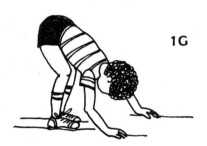 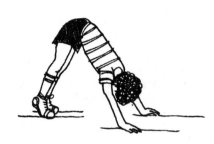

1G

CRAB WALK
Inverted body position on hands and feet with stomach pointed to the ceiling. (See previous illustration 1C on page 33.)

ACTIVITY – 2 – LOCOMOTOR PRACTICE

Walk, run, jump and hop. Have students first walk slowly around the room. Ask them to jog slowly around the room being careful not to bump into anyone. In a straight line ask the group to jump on two feet forward to you. Then ask them to jump backwards to where they began. Repeat this, asking students to do the same, while this time hopping on one foot and then the other. (These techniques are often enhanced with the instructor standing in the center and beating a drum in time with each locomotor movement.)

ACTIVITY – 3 – LOCOMOTOR PRACTICE

Skip, gallop, slide and leap. Start by introducing the gallop and how to change the lead foot. Give students a lot of practice at switching their lead foot before you introduce skipping. Have students switch on a given command. Increase the frequency of times that you ask students to change their lead foot until they are skipping. This is the easiest teaching progression for teaching skipping. (Children generally do not learn to skip until they are 5 years old.) Practice all locomotor skills performing them going forward, sideways and backwards.

ACTIVITY – 4 – HOPPING IN HOOPS

Children enjoy the challenge of hopping a pattern using hoops lined up in an unpredictable pattern.

ACTIVITY – 5 – HOPPING AND JUMPING IN PATTERNS

Practice hopping and jumping using ropes laid out which look like a tic tac toe. Ask students to jump a certain pattern. For example, jump forward 3 times and sideways one time. Or jump forward, backward and across. As well as a sequencing task, this also reinforces locomotor skills.

ACTIVITY – 6 – HOPPING

Can you take off and land on one foot? Can you take off on one foot and land on the other? Can you jump on 2 feet? Can you hop in place on one foot? Can you hop forward? Now try the other foot. Everyone hop forward around a circle formation and change to the other foot. Can you hop backwards? Sideways?

ACTIVITY – 7 – LOCOMOTOR MOVEMENTS

Practice locomotor movements on a track laid out around the room. Use plastic numbers or the alphabet. If you are outside on the blacktop, you can even use colored chalk and write in any number of commands or formations. An alphabet trail is most appropriate for kindergartens and pre-schools. A number track is also useful in assisting children in learning their numbers while at the same time practicing a locomotor skill.

ACTIVITY – 8 – PATHWAYS

Draw a variety of colored chalk pathways on the blacktop (one per child). Play music and have children practice a designed loco-motor skill while moving from one end of their pathway to the other. On the signal (whistle), have them move to a new pathway and practice a different locomotor skill.

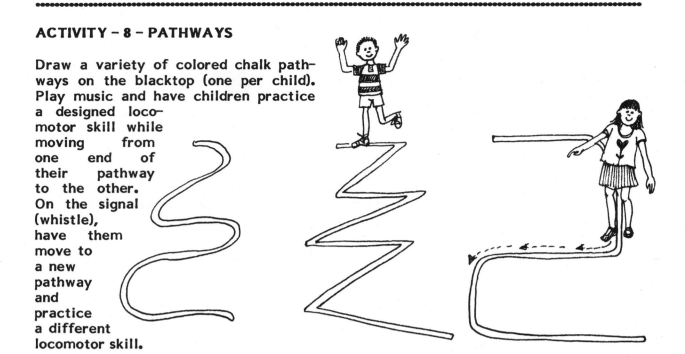

ACTIVITY – 9 – LOCOMOTOR SKILLS WITH PARACHUTE

Lay the parachute out on the ground. Ask students to practice jogging, walking backward, sliding, skipping, hopping and jumping in different directions (that is, forward, backwards or sideways around the parachute). Note: This is a good opportunity to evaluate children's locomotor abilities.

ACTIVITY – 10 – NUMBER EXCHANGE WITH PARACHUTE

Have students number off by fours around the parachute. Then, as we raise the chute, the teacher calls out a number and a locomotor skill. The children with that number proceed under the chute and across to the other side doing the designated skill. To make it into a fun game, allow the children to pull the chute down quickly, trying to capture people inside, if you call "running". Otherwise, allow the chute to collapse naturally.

ACTIVITY – 11 – MUSICAL HOOPS

This game is a takeoff on "musical chairs" (one less hoop than the number of children in the class). The person in the middle calls out a locomotor skill and the music starts. The other children around the circle must keep moving, performing the locomotor skill called out until the music stops. At that time each student scrambles for a hoop. The person without a hoop goes to the middle and the game continues.

●●

ACTIVITY - 12 - HILL DILL GAME

One child is selected to be "it" standing between parallel lines spaced widely apart. The remaining children are lined up side by side on one parallel line. The person who is "it" chants: "Hill dill, come over the hill before I catch you standing still". On the word "still", all the children run, attempting to get to the opposite parallel line without getting tagged. Those who are tagged become "it" also. Those who are "it" repeat the chant and the game continues. Game could be modified to include other locomotor skills besides running.

●●

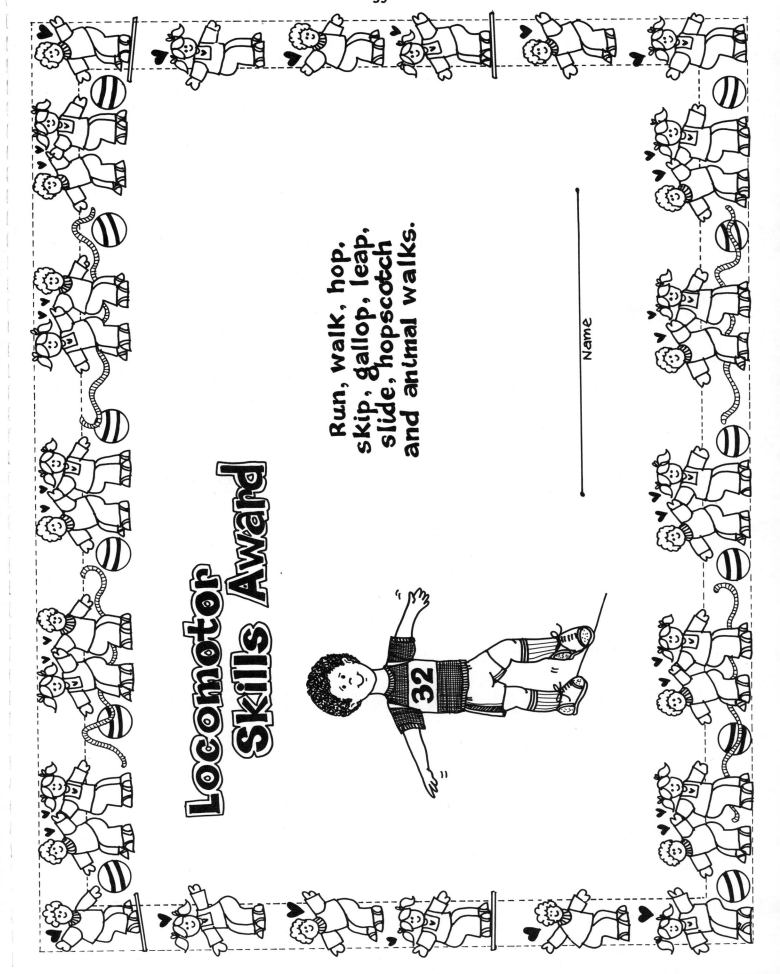

Locomotor Skills Award

Run, walk, hop, skip, gallop, leap, slide, hopscotch and animal walks.

Name

Chapter 6

HAND-EYE COORDINATION

OBJECTIVES

1) Each student will learn an overhand throw.

2) Each student will be instructed in an underhand throw.

3) Each student will be instructed in a drop and catch sequence.

4) Each student will learn the techniques of throwing a nerf frisbee.

5) Students will be instructed in dribbling techniques.

6) Each student will be instructed on correct catching techniques.

EQUIPMENT NEEDS

Playground rubber ball 8" diameter, nerf balls of varying sizes, frisbee, bean bags, milk carton scoops, ring toss games, beach balls, hoops, clothespins and blocks.

INSTRUCTIONAL TIPS

1) A dominate or preferred hand is generally evident after 5 years of age. Children, nevertheless, should be encouraged to do all activities using both hands.

2) Hand-eye coordination is the cornerstone of basic sports skill development.

3) Emphasize that correct form is more important than accuracy when practicing throwing skills.

4) When introducing catching techniques, use a nerf or beach ball for children who display fear.

ACTIVITY – 1 – DROP AND CATCH PLAYGROUND BALLS

Have each student sit inside a hula hoop holding a red playground ball. Demonstrate how to stand with your feet outside the hoop and drop and catch the ball 5 times. (When a child can consistently drop and catch the ball 5 times without missing, he is ready to be instructed in dribbling.)

ACTIVITY - 2 - OVERHAND THROWING BEAN BAGS

Have each student sit in a line behind their bean bag. Demonstrate an overhand throw. Throw bean bag at a very large target to insure success. A student who can successfully throw and hit a target 5 times in a row is ready for one giant step backwards. Have students, one at a time, throw their bean bags to you. Check to see that their technique is correct. (See illustration.)

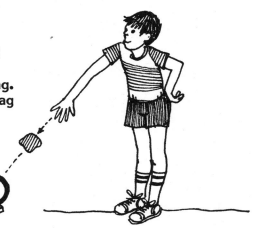

ACTIVITY - 3 - UNDERHAND THROWING BEAN BAGS

Same as for Activity 2 only use the underhand technique. (See illustration.)

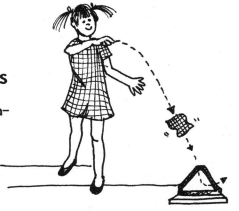

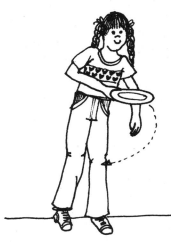

ACTIVITY - 4 - NERF FRISBEES

Each student should have a nerf frisbee. Show them the correct technique for throwing a frisbee. Have each student try and throw their frisbee through one of several wooden (cardboard, etc.) shapes. (See illustration.)

ACTIVITY – 5 – DRIBBLING PLAYGROUND BALLS

A student should not attempt to dribble a ball until he is proficient at the bounce and catch sequence given in Activity 1 on page 40. Dribbling is always with one hand and should be taught as such. Emphasize using ones' finger tips and not slapping the ball. Dribble for 10 times consistently with each hand while stationary, before attempting to dribble while moving forward. (See illustration.)

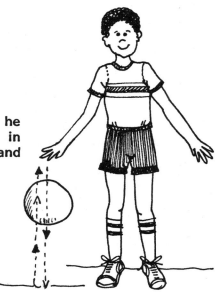

ACTIVITY – 6 – CATCHING BEAN BAGS

Demonstrate to all students the correct technique for catching an object. Emphasize that both hands should be used! Have students "give" with an object as it approaches their hands. Tracking or keeping their eyes on the object is equally important. (See illustration.)

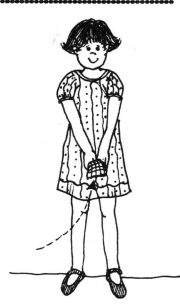

ACTIVITY – 7 – THROWING AND CATCHING NERF BALLS

A variety of sizes and weights are the best. (See illustration.) Have students try first to throw the ball above their heads and catch it. Have them throw it above their heads and catch it 5 times without moving their feet. With partners: Have students pick a partner and practice throwing and catching with that partner from a relatively close distance in the beginning and moving farther apart as their skills improve.

ACTIVITY – 8 – THROWING AND CATCHING SCOOPS

Give each student a scoop and a bean bag. (See illustration.) Have them practice throwing the bean bag above their heads and catching it in the scoop. Partners: Have each student throw and catch using the scoops and bean bags with a friend.

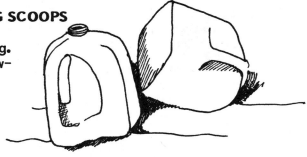

ACTIVITY – 9 – THROWING RINGS

Have students start out by throwing the rings into a hula hoop to insure success. As students get better skilled, keep decreasing the size of the target until they can use the regular "ring toss" pole. (Throwing rings to land around a pole.)

ACTIVITY – 10 – CATCHING SMALL PLAYGROUND BALLS

Have students practice throwing the ball above their heads and see if they can clap their hands before they catch it. Increase the number of claps.

ACTIVITY – 11 – BATTING OR HITTING BEACH BALLS

Let one student stand in the middle of the circle. Have her bat the beach ball up into the air with her hands while calling the name of a child in the circle. The selected child must come to the center of the circle and catch the beach ball before it touches the ground.

ACTIVITY – 12 – RING TOSS GAME WITH HOOPS AND BEAN BAGS

Put a plastic number inside each hoop to indicate points earned for landing in the hoop. If able, have students play the game by keeping score of the points they have earned by throwing the bean bags into the hoops.

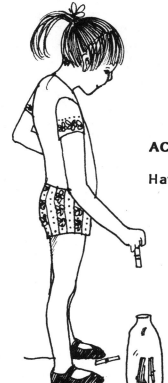

ACTIVITY – 13 – BUCKET AND CLOTHESPINS GAME

Have students try to drop the clothespins into a bucket or jar
    by standing over it and holding the clothespins waist high.
    (See illustration.)

ACTIVITY – 14 – DODGEBALL WITH PLAYGROUND BALL

Make a circle. Have one student in the middle. Let students throw or roll the ball
and try to hit the student in the middle.

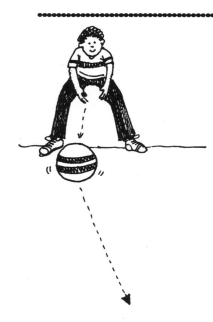

ACTIVITY – 15 – BOWLING WITH SMALL PLAYGROUND BALL AND BLOCKS

Set up approximately 5 small blocks for each group. Have
one student at a time roll a playground ball and try to
knock over the blocks. (See illustration.) Adjust the distance (closer for those children who have difficulty and
farther back for those children who achieve early success
with this activity).

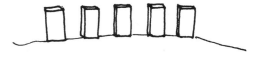

ACTIVITY - 16 - TARGET BOUNCE WITH BEAN BAG AND PLAYGROUND BALL

Put a bean bag on the floor. Two players bounce the ball back and forth to each other trying to bounce the ball on the bean bag. (See illustration.) Every time the bean bag is hit, the player responsible would get a point. Game is to see who can get to 10 first. If bean bag is too large and easy to hit, use a smaller object like a penny.

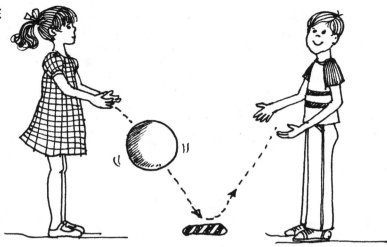

MORE BALL ACTIVITIES

The following activities are for those who would like more concentrated hand-eye coordination activities using that ever popular playground equipment item, namely, the "ball". Each of the 3 ball activities (Exploration, Throwing & Catching With Partner, and Dribbling) are written progressively for greater skill development.

ACTIVITY - 17 - EXPLORATION

1) Bounce and catch (2 hands).
2) Toss above head and catch.
3) Toss above head - let bounce - and catch.
4) Toss above head - let bounce - turn and catch.
5) Bounce, clap hands, and catch.
6) Roll ball - run and field it.
7) Run - toss ball in air and catch it.
8) Bounce under each leg and catch it.
9) Jump over ball (forward and backward).
10) Toss ball from hand to hand.
11) Bounce ball waist high (head high, knee high).
12) Bounce ball lightly (strongly).
13) Bounce ball and catch it low (catch it high).

ACTIVITY – 18 – THROWING AND CATCHING WITH PARTNER

1) Underhand toss to partner (two hands).
2) Underhand toss to partner (one hand).
3) Overhand toss to partner (two hands chest pass).
4) Overhand toss to partner (one hand).
5) Bounce pass to partner (two hands).
6) Bounce pass to partner (one hand).
7) Underhand high toss to partner (preferred hand).

ACTIVITY – 19 – DRIBBLING

1) Bounce and catch (2 hands).
2) Two hand dribble.
3) Preferred hand dribble (in place).
4) Dribble low and dribble high (in place).
5) Least preferred hand dribble (in place).
6) Walk and dribble.
7) Changing hands dribble (in place).
8) Walk and dribble changing hands.
9) Run and dribble (either hand).
10) Stop and go dribbling.

HAND-EYE CHECKLIST	Overhand Throw	Underhand Throw	Drop And Catch Sequence	Throw A Frisbee	Dribble 10 Times	Catch With Hands	Tracks Object						
NAME					– 47 –								

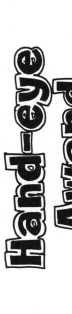

Hand-eye Award

Overhand and underhand throwing, dribbling, catching, tracking an object, and throwing a frisbee.

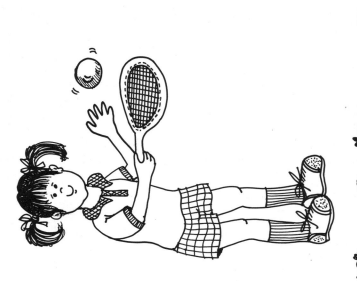

Name

Chapter 7

SOCIAL SKILL DEVELOPMENT THROUGH PARACHUTE ACTIVITIES

OBJECTIVES

1) Students will interact appropriately with peers.

2) Students will follow verbal directions so as to accomplish group goals.

3) Students will wait patiently for their turn.

4) Students will participate for the duration of the activity.

5) Students will return equipment neatly.

EQUIPMENT NEEDS

Parachute for all activities, bean bags, balls and jump ropes.

INSTRUCTIONAL TIPS

1) Encourage cooperation. Inform children that parachute activities may be accomplished only if everyone works together.

2) When giving instructions, it is best to have children sitting with legs crossed and the parachute pulled taunt.

3) Parachute play is enjoyed by both preschool and elementary school children.

4) It is important that the teacher instructs students in the vocabulary of the parachute. Some recommended commands are: "Inflate, deflate, ready—begin, and pull the parachute tight and hold it on the ground".

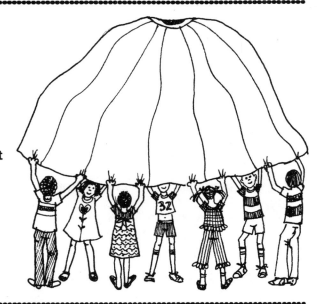

ACTIVITY – 1 – SHAKE THE RUG

Shake the parachute waist high, chest high, and above the head (see illustration).

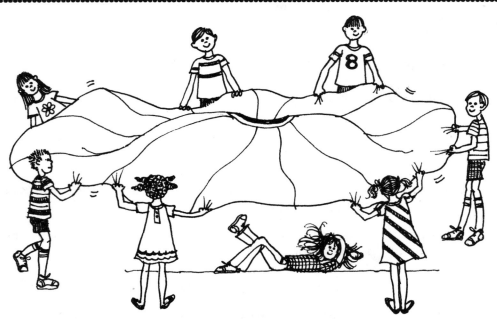

ACTIVITY – 2 – MAKE WIND

Quick up and down movements in unison. Have some students lie under parachute to feel the wind.

ACTIVITY – 3 – BILLOW A CLOUD

Billow parachute high above head.

ACTIVITY – 4 – TOSS A CLOUD

Billow the parachute high and on the count of 3, release the parachute. When it is released in unison it will float to the ceiling.

ACTIVITY – 5 – CIRCLE THE CHUTE

Place a large ball on the parachute and coordinate up and down movements of the chute to make the ball roll around the perimeter. (See illustration.)

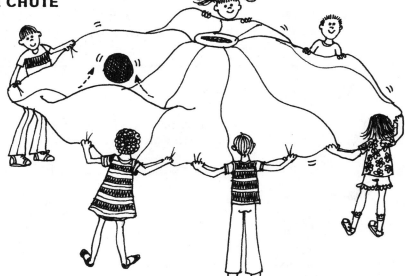

ACTIVITY – 6 – TOSS A BALL

Place a large ball on the chute and in unison toss it into the air and catch it on the chute. (See illustration.)

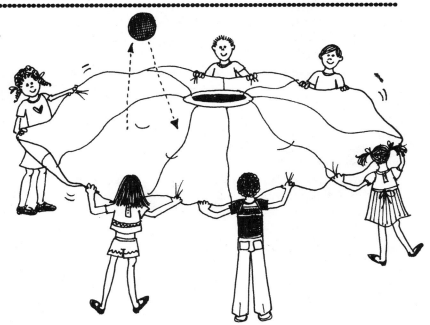

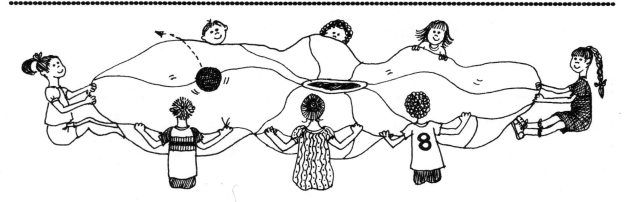

ACTIVITY – 7 – OCEAN WAVES

Ripple the chute to simulate ocean waves. Place a ball on the chute and attempt to make the ball go off the chute by someone else. (See illustration.)

ACTIVITY – 8 – GHOST CITY

Select 10 to 15 students to assume a static position of their choice. Billow the chute above them and then let it settle down over them.

ACTIVITY – 9 – DRAGON

Children run with parachute billowing behind them.

ACTIVITY – 10 – CHUTE TRAP

While the chute is being held taunt by about half the class, have the other half run or crawl under the chute. On a signal, kids let go and try to trap people inside.

ACTIVITY – 11 – POPCORN

Put balls and bean bags on the chute and make waves while trying to keep all the corn (balls and bean bags) on the parachute. (See illustration.)

ACTIVITY – 12 – SNAKE PIT

Put jump ropes on the parachute. Have the children make waves while being careful not to get bitten by a "snake". (See illustration.)

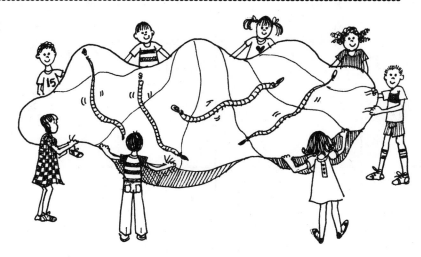

MORE PARACHUTE ACTIVITIES FOR OLDER CHILDREN

ACTIVITY – 13 – NUMBER EXCHANGE

Have students number off in a 1, 2, 3, 4, 5, 6/1, 2, 3, 4, 5, 6 pattern. When the students have inflated the parachute as high as possible, call out a number. Everyone with that number lets go of the chute, ducks quickly under it, and exchanges places with another person having the same number. Students on the outside let go of the chute and try to catch students inside.

ACTIVITY – 14 – FOX AND THE SQUIRREL

All students are seated Indian style around the chute. One child becomes the squirrel and crawls on his hands and knees under the chute while all the other children make waves while sitting. Select one other child to crawl on top and try to catch the squirrel. When the squirrel is caught, two new people are selected.

ACTIVITY – 15 – HOLE IN ONE

Use balls that are two different colors. Divide group into two equal teams on opposite sides of the parachute. The object of the game is to shake the other's balls into the hole in the middle of the chute.

SOCIAL SKILL DEVELOPMENT CHECKLIST NAME	Follows Directions	Waits Turn	Cooperates With Peers	Participates Willingly	Cares For Equipment	Returns Equipment	Displays Good Sportsmanship							

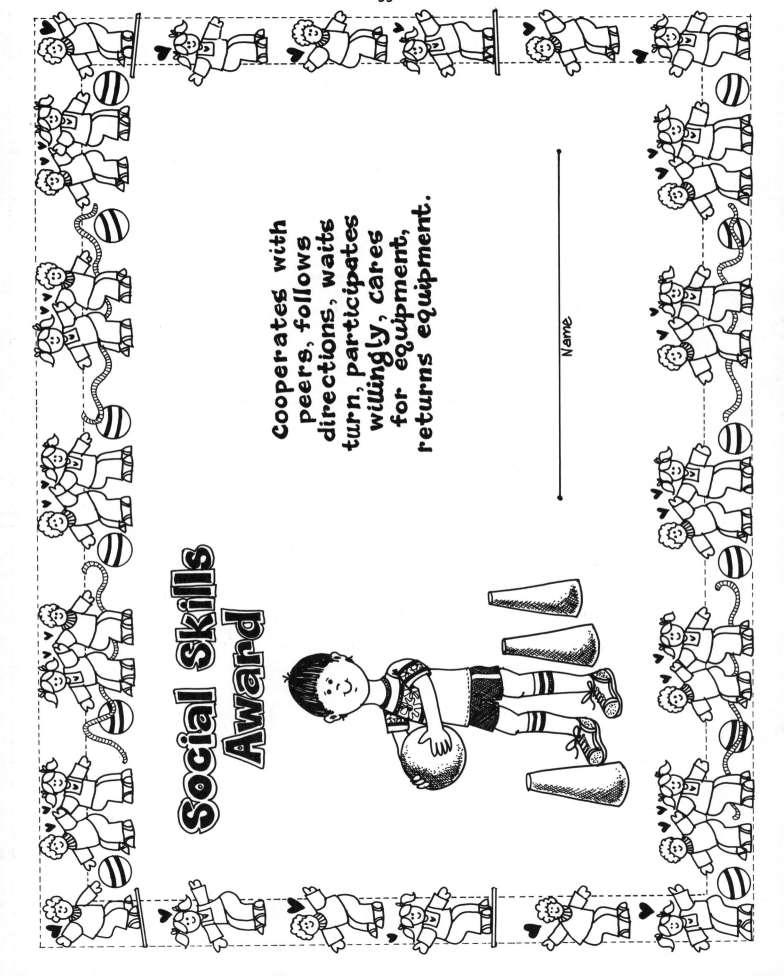

Social Skills Award

Cooperates with peers, follows directions, waits turn, participates willingly, cares for equipment, returns equipment.

Name

NAME	Walk – Smoothly	Run Alternating Arm Movement	Hop Left & Right	Jump Two Feet	Skip	Gallop	Slide	Animal Walks	Pathways	Hop Scotch			

LOCOMOTOR CHECKLIST

Chapter 8

SMALL MOTOR COORDINATION

OBJECTIVES

1) Each student will string a lacing board.

2) Each Student will learn to string beads.

3) Each student will learn to put clothespins on the side of a can.

4) Each student will touch each finger to the thumb.

5) Each student will demonstrate the "open-close fingers" game.

6) Each student will sort and arrange the perceptual shapes by color.

7) Each student will demonstrate finger manipulative activities with rhythm sticks.

8) Students will demonstrate peg board abilities.

EQUIPMENT NEEDS

Lacing board, beads, clothespins, vinyl shapes, rhythm sticks and peg boards.

INSTRUCTIONAL TIPS

Students vary greatly in their small motor abilities. Adequate time should be devoted to each activity to insure that students do not become anxious or fatigued.

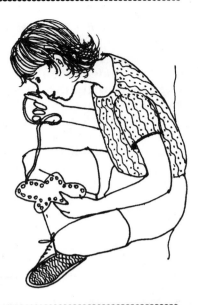

ACTIVITY – 1 – LACING BOARD

Each student should receive a lacing board to practice with at his own pace. Have students thread and unthread their own work. (See illustration.)

ACTIVITY – 2 – BEAD STRINGING

Stringing beads is a wonderful fine motor activity which allows for cognitive skill development as well. Have students string and unstring their beads. Have students count the number of beads they were given. Have them arrange their beads by color into piles. Have them sort their beads by shape. Have students organize their beads from largest to smallest. Discuss the above listed activities. Give each student a pattern to follow. An example might be a color pattern or a shape pattern. Start with a pattern of 2 and work up.

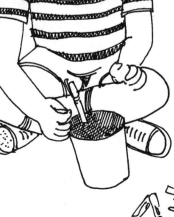

ACTIVITY – 3 – CLOTHESPINS

Have the students put the clothespins on the side of a lid, jar or can. (See illustration.) A young child will lack finger strength and dexterity; therefore allow him to use both hands to open the clothespins. An older child can use only one hand and should be encouraged to put his other hand behind his back while doing this activity. (See Activity 2 for cognitive suggestions and progressions.)

ACTIVITY – 4 – TOUCH THE FINGERS INDEPENDENTLY

The child is to touch all the finger tips of one hand in succession, independently, with the thumb of the same hand beginning with the little finger. The child then repeats the task in reverse order, starting with the index finger. (See illustration.) Say, "Let me see you touch your finger tips with your thumb." "Start with your little finger and touch each finger like this. Then go back again to your little finger." Demonstrate.

ACTIVITY – 5 – OPEN AND CLOSE FINGERS

Child should start with both hands closed into fists. Have students repeat and act out the song. "Open shut them, open shut them, give a little clap! Open shut them, open shut them, put them in your lap." An advanced version of this activity is to ask students to open one hand while at the same time closing the other.

ACTIVITY – 6 – SHAPES

Using small geometric shapes that the students know, ask them to sort the shapes into stacks. Ask them to line up shapes from the smallest to the largest. (See illustration.) Ask them to arrange the shapes by color. Take the time to also talk about the first and last shape in their line. Which group has more or less, or which ones are the same or different.

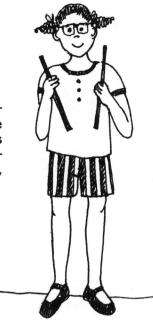

ACTIVITY – 7 – RHYTHM STICKS

Rhythm sticks can be used for a fine motor activity emphasizing finger control and dexterity by: rolling them like a log in front of you, climbing up the sticks with your fingers as if you were a spider, hammering the sticks on end, dropping one stick and catching it before it hits the ground, flipping a stick, twirling a stick, etc. (See illustration.)

ACTIVITY – 8 – PEG BOARDS

Peg boards can be used in the same manner as many of those activities described in Activity 2 on page 57. (See illustration.)

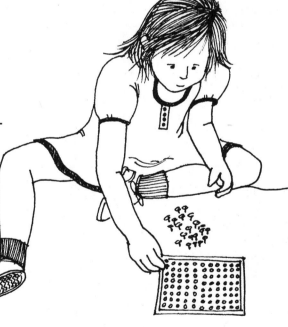

SMALL MOTOR COOR-DINATION CHECKLIST NAME	Lace Board	Bead Stringing	Clothespins	Touch Finger Tips	Open And Close Hands	Sort Shapes Size, Color, Etc.	Finger Manipulatives	Peg Boards					
						– 60 –							

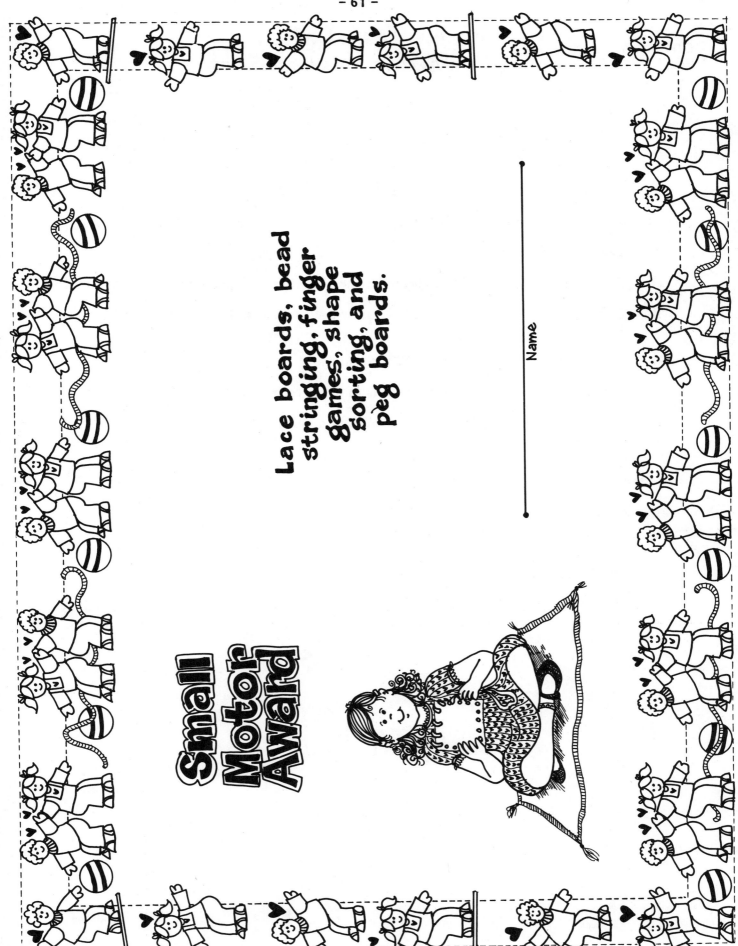

Lace boards, bead stringing, finger games, shape sorting, and peg boards.

Name

Small Motor Award

Chapter 9

SKILL DEVELOPMENT THROUGH GAMES

OBJECTIVES

Each of the following objectives can be accomplished in a game setting.

1)   Each student should practice rolling a ball to a target.

2)   Each student should exhibit throwing and catching techniques in a game setting.

3)   Each student should catch a playground ball on the first bounce when reacting to their name.

4)   Students will practice auditory discrimination.

5)   Students will exhibit locomotor skills in game formats.

6)   Students will exhibit kicking techniques in a game setting.

EQUIPMENT NEEDS

Playground ball 8" in diameter, soccer type ball, nerf ball, hoops, and music.

INSTRUCTIONAL TIPS

An easy and efficient way to test children is by using a checklist while observing the desired skill during a game situation. Children are relaxed and having fun, making the testing situation stress free.

HAND-EYE COORDINATION

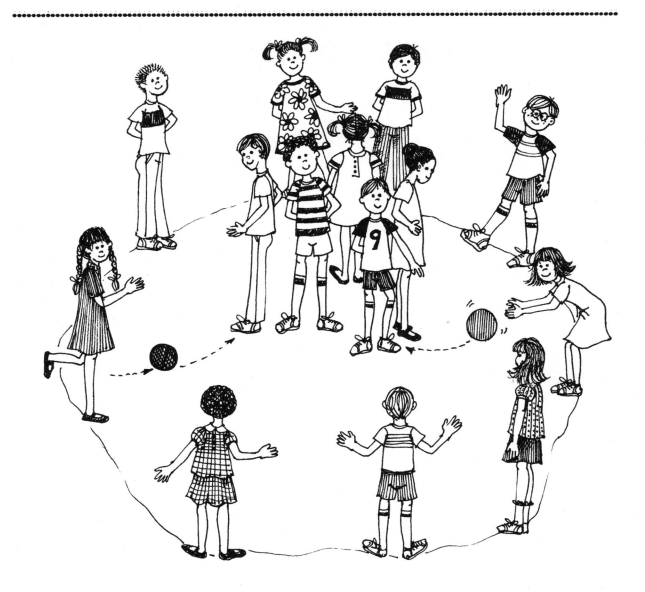

ACTIVITY – 1 – BOWLING DODGEBALL

Players are lined up around a circle. Select 5 players to be in the center representing the stationary "pins". Circle players attempt to put the center players out by rolling a playground ball and hitting them. (See illustration.) When a player is hit, he changes places with the circle player who hit him. Keep 2 to 3 balls going for more movement activity.

ACTIVITY – 2 – PIN BALL DODGEBALL

Same format as bowling dodgeball except that circle players try to roll the playground ball through a center player's legs.

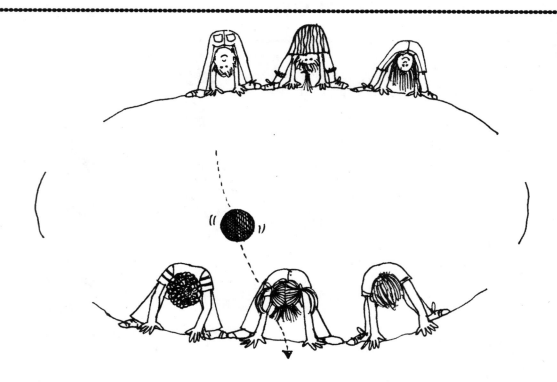

ACTIVITY - 3 - ADVANCED GROUP BOWLING

All players form a circle, straddling their feet so that they are spread apart and touching the players' feet next to them. All players then turn around backwards, bend over and look through their legs. Object is to send the playground ball through a player's legs before he can get his hands down and stop it. Players must keep their hands on their knees until the ball is rolled at them. Another game version is that the players can keep their hands down by their ankles or feet until the ball is rolled at them as shown in the illustration.

ACTIVITY - 4 - ROUNDERS

Players are divided into 2 teams. One team is "UP" at home plate and the other team takes the bases with the remaining players scattered out in the field. The teacher says, "GO" and the first runner throws a playground size ball and starts running. It is a race to see which (runner or ball) gets around the bases and home first. If the runner wins, then he scores a point. All players get to throw and run once, then the whole team switches with the opposing team. The team with the most points at the end of the time period wins. The opposing field team retrieves the ball and throws it to first base, then around the other bases, in sequence, to home. It is advised that the ball be thrown one time around the bases to the runner's home plate (2 times around for younger children). Advanced students will want to use a smaller ball and it is advised that the field team throws the ball 2 times around the bases to the runner's one run around to home plate. (See illustration at the top of page 65.)

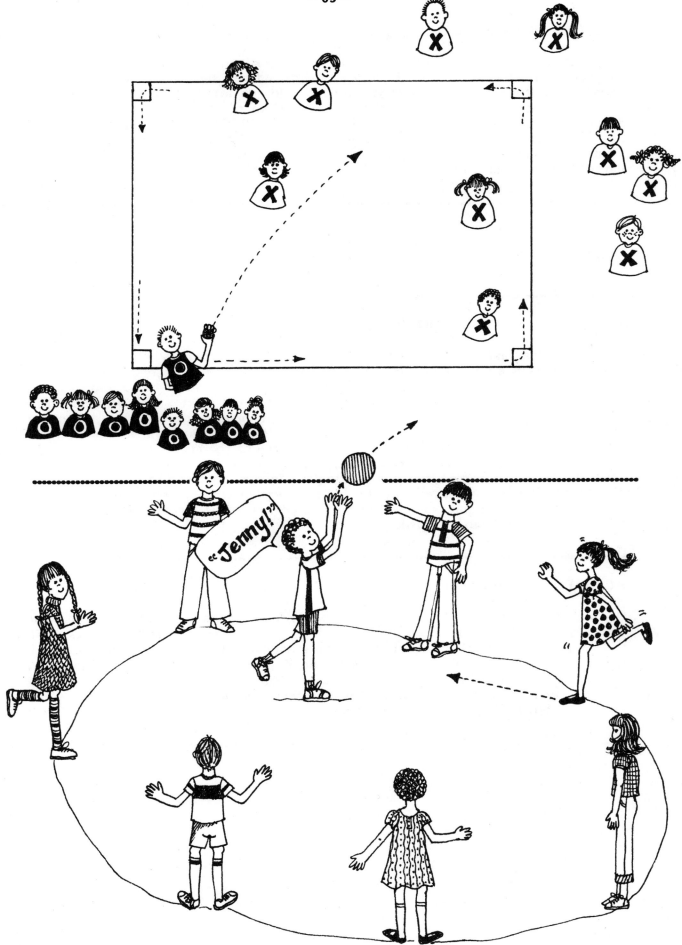

"Jenny!"

ACTIVITY - 5 - NAME BALL

All students stand around a circle. The teacher instructs one student to be "it" in the center of the circle. "It" throws a playground ball up into the air and calls a name. The student whose name is called should run into the center of the circle and catch the ball. (See illustration at the bottom of page 65.) Preschoolers will need at least 2 bounces. Kindergarten students will usually need one bounce and other children, in time, will progress to no bounces. The child whose name is called would then become the center player whether or not she retrieves the ball by catching it in the appropriate manner.

LOCOMOTOR

ACTIVITY - 6 - MUSICAL HOOPS

This game is a takeoff on musical chairs. Instead of chairs, hula hoops are arranged in a circle with a person in the center of each hoop. (There is one less hoop than the number of children in the game.) A person in the middle of the circle of hoops calls out a locomotor skill and the music (your choice) starts. The other children around the circle must keep moving from hoop to hoop performing the locomotor skill called out until the music stops. At that time, each student scrambles for a hoop. The person without a hoop goes to the middle of the hoop circle and the game continues. (In one version of the game, the person in the center of the circle of hoops is the extra person and can participate in moving from hoop to hoop as he calls out a locomotor movement. In another version, the person in the center of the hoop circle stays put while another extra person in the circle tries to find their own hoop when the music stops.)

ACTIVITY - 7 - HILL DILL

One child is selected to be "it" and stands between 2 parallel lines. The remaining children are lined up side by side on one line. The person who is "it" chants, "Hill Dill come over the hill before I catch you standing still". On the word "still", all the children run (gallop) to the opposite end line attempting not to get tagged by "it". Those who are tagged become "it" also. Those who are "it" repeat the chant together and the game continues. The game should be modified to include other locomotor skills besides running (galloping).

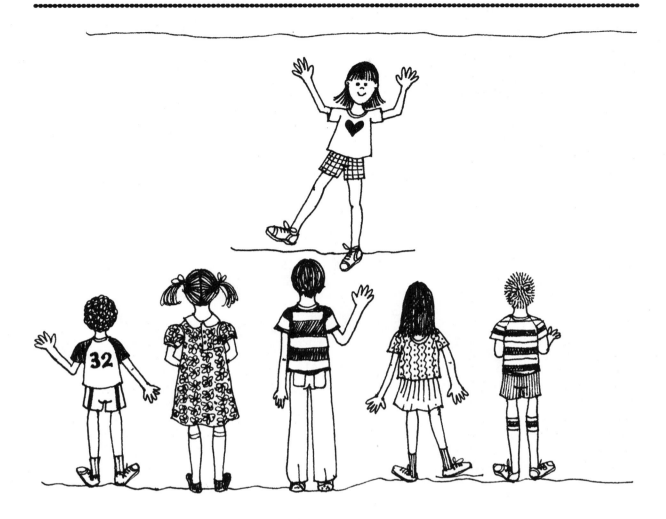

ACTIVITY – 8 – MAN FROM MARS

This game requires 2 lines spread approximately 50 feet apart. All players line up on one of the lines. A student is selected to be the "Man From Mars" and he stands in the center of the 2 lines. (See illustration.) All players call, "Man From Mars, Man From Mars. Will you take us to the stars?" All students then take off for the other line while performing a locomotor pattern of their choice. "Man From Mars" replies, "Only if you are skipping". Those who are performing the locomotor pattern called may continue safely to the other line. The other students must continue heading for the other line with the possibility of being tagged. All who are tagged must help the "Man From Mars" and the game continues. Object is to be the last one tagged.

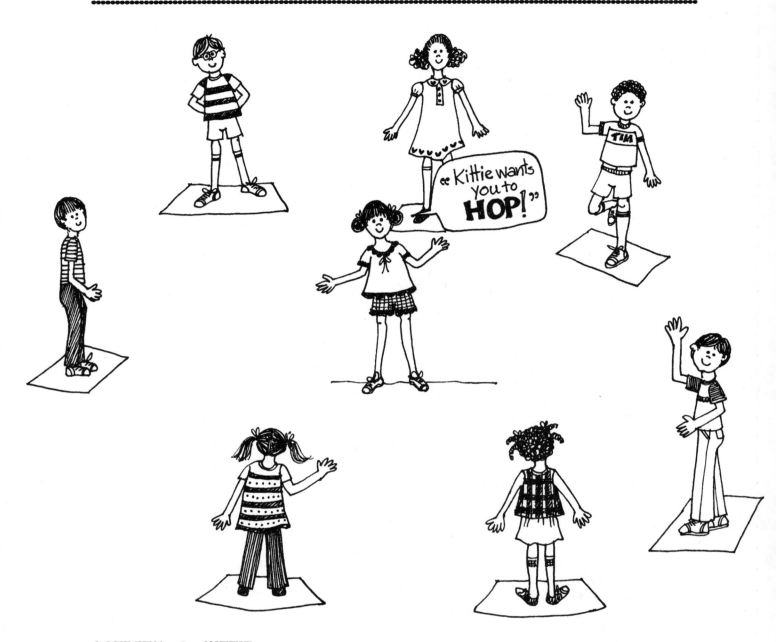

ACTIVITY – 9 – KITTIE

Each child is given a carpet to stand on. The carpets should be laid out to form a large circle. One child is asked to be the "Kittie" and stand in the center. The "Kittie" begins play by saying, "Kittie wants you to_____ ". (Fill in the name of a locomotor skill.) (See illustration.) When a skill is called, all the players (including "Kittie") must use the locomotor skill called and go to a new carpet. One child will be without a carpet and should then take his place in the center as "Kittie" and the game continues. The object of the game is to not get stuck in the middle.

EYE-FOOT GAMES

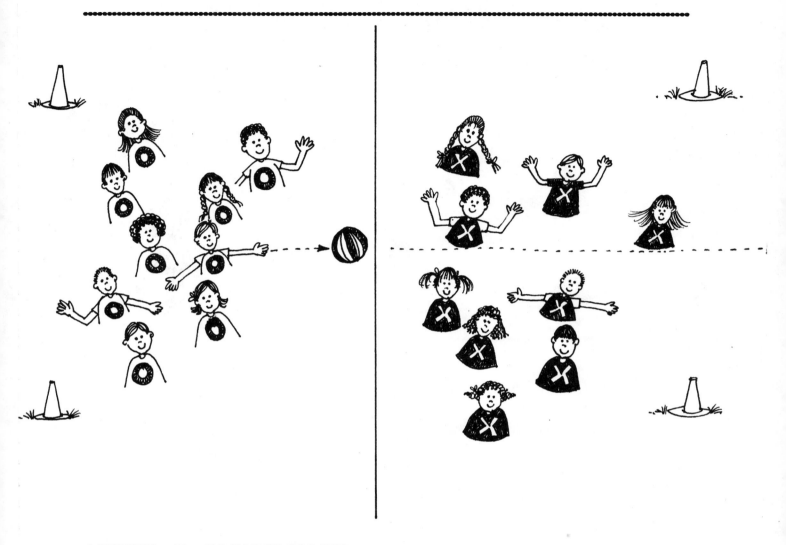

ACTIVITY – 10 – GO FOR IT SOCCER

Players should be divided into 2 teams. A soccer ball or playground ball is placed in the center of a dividing line to start play. Two game cones should be placed for a goal at each end of a playing area (four cones total). (Side lines and end lines are not necessary.) Students from both teams try to score by kicking the ball through their respective goals. The only rule is that the ball must go through a goal from the correct direction. (See illustration.) Game continues until someone scores. You may keep score, if you wish, or start a new game and play for "fun" each time.

ACTIVITY – 11 – CIRCLE SOCCER

Players line up around the circle. A line cutting the circle is drawn to separate the 2 teams. The object is to kick a soccer ball past an opponent and out of the circle. (The ball should always be kicked below waist level.) (See illustration at the top of page 70.) One point is awarded for each goal. Players can block or trap the ball with any part of their bodies except their hands and arms. Students may use more than one soccer ball.

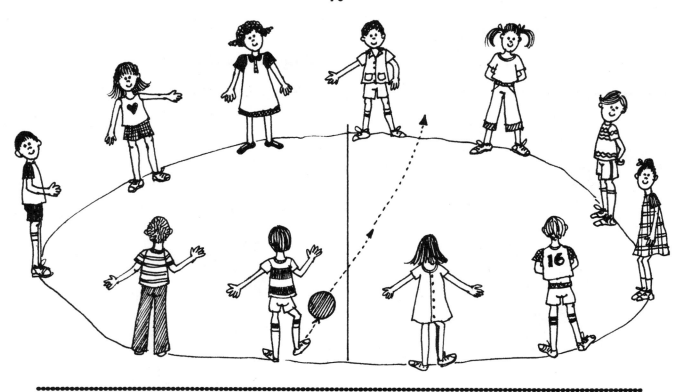

BALANCE

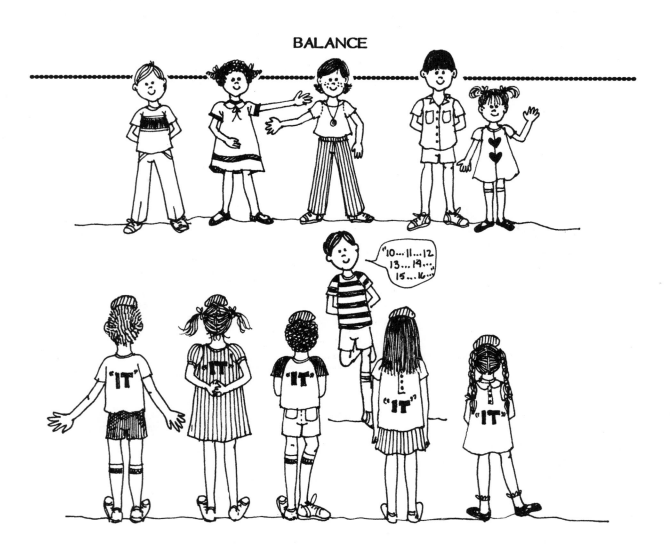

ACTIVITY - 12 - BEAN BAG STUCK IN THE MUD

Four or more players are selected to be "it". Their mission is to balance a bean bag on their (heads, hands, shoulders, etc.) while trying to tag regular players and stop the action (tagged players freeze in position). Once a player is tagged, he must stay in one spot (freeze) and balance on one foot and count to 25 out-loud. If all players are not frozen when previously tagged players finish their count, the tagged (frozen) players can unfreeze after their count is up and may again move around to avoid being tagged anew and the game continues. When all players are "frozen", the 4 or more new taggers are selected for the next game! (For clarity, the illustration at the bottom of page 70, artificially separates out the different states the players are in, that is, a group of "its" with bean bags on their heads, a tagged player counting to 25, and a group of untagged players. In reality, all the "its" would be running after the untagged players within a confined area.)

●●●

SKILL DEVELOP-MENT THRU GAMES CHECKLIST NAME	Bowling Games Rolling To Target	Rounders Throwing And Catching	Name Ball Catching (On Bounce)	Musical Hoops Locomotor Skill	Hill Dill Locomotor Skill	Man From Mars Locomotor Skill	Kittie Locomotor Skill	Soccer Kicking	Bean Bag Balancing				

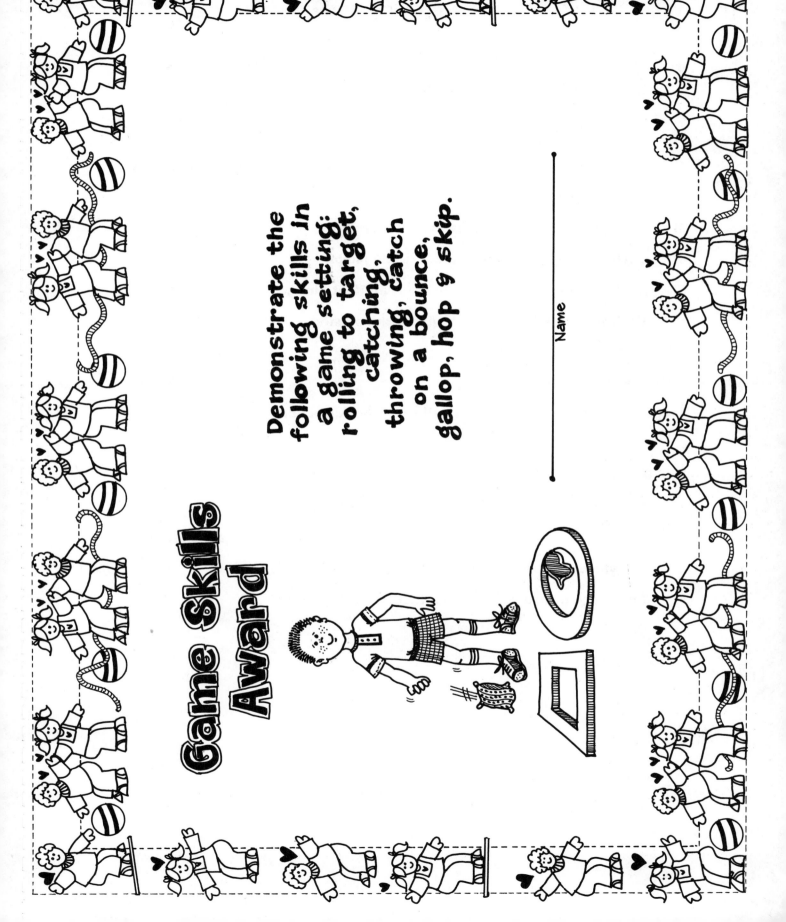

Game Skills Award

Demonstrate the following skills in a game setting: rolling to target, catching, throwing, catch on a bounce, gallop, hop & skip.

Name

Chapter 10

TOTAL BODY COORDINATION

OBJECTIVES

1) Students will learn to jump up and down on a jogger 10 times rhythmically.

2) Each student will learn a half turn.

3) Each student will learn cross lateral marching.

4) Each student will demonstrate straddle jumps.

5) Each student will demonstrate alternate feet kicks.

6) Each student will sequence multiple skills listed above.

EQUIPMENT NEEDS

Jogger. (Sometimes known as a small exercise trampoline.)

INSTRUCTIONAL TIPS

1) Hold the child's hands at all times when on the jogger.

2) Short turns are best. Children generally tire after about 30 seconds.

3) Ask students to jump only in the center of the jogger.

4) Encourage controlled jumping. Discourage high jumping.

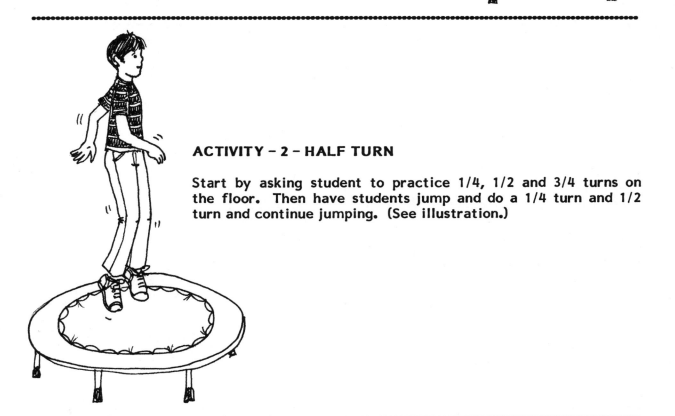

ACTIVITY – 1 – RHYTHMIC JUMPING

Have student jump with 2 feet up into the air, getting the feel of the jogger. (See illustration.) Ask students to jump 10 times and then stop and bend knees to come to a controlled stop. Students should always be assisted when getting off the jogger. Ask them to step off. Never jump off, as they might get injured.

ACTIVITY – 2 – HALF TURN

Start by asking student to practice 1/4, 1/2 and 3/4 turns on the floor. Then have students jump and do a 1/4 turn and 1/2 turn and continue jumping. (See illustration.)

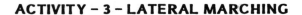

ACTIVITY – 3 – LATERAL MARCHING

Have students experience marching on the jogger. Have them try to hop on one foot. Have them try to develop a rhythm with marching and jumping. (See illustration.)

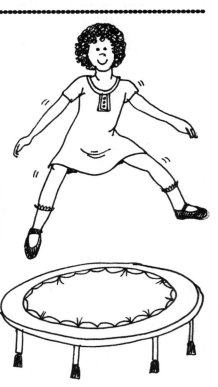

ACTIVITY – 4 – STRADDLE JUMPS

Have students jump on the floor with their legs spread and extended in front of them (straddle jump). Ask them to then do a straddle jump on the jogger. (See illustration.) Younger students should be encouraged to simply spread their legs to the side and back.

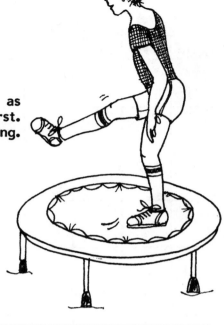

ACTIVITY – 5 – ALTERNATE FEET KICKS

Alternate feet kick forward, trying to keep the legs as straight as possible in front of them on the floor first. Then move the student to the jogger to try the same thing. (See illustration.)

ACTIVITY – 6 – SEQUENCING OF MULTIPLE SKILLS

Have students jump 3 times and then do a 1/2 turn followed by a straddle jump. Then continue jumping and once they can do this simple sequence satisfactorily, add still more skills to the sequence in the following progression: bouncing (jumping), 1/2 turn, cross lateral marching, straddle jumps, and alternate feet kicks. Mix up the sequence.

TOTAL BODY COORDINATION CHECKLIST NAME	Rhythmic Jumping	Cross Lateral Marching	Straddle Jumps	½ Turn	Alternate Kicks	Sequencing Of Multiple Skills – 78 –									

coordination Award

Rhythmic jumping, cross lateral marching, straddle jumps, 1/2 turns, and sequencing of multiple skills.

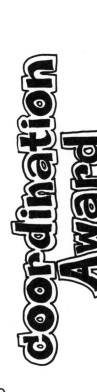

Name

EQUIPMENT RECOMMENDATIONS

Below are listed equipment items needed for a perceptual-motor type program as described in this book. For optimal results in your own program, use specific equipment sizes when specified.

Equipment Item	Quantity Needed	Size Specified (If Any)
Walking Board	1	8 ft
Balance Board	2	
Blocks	1 set	
Bean Bags	15	
Coordination Ladder	1	
Tin Can Stilts	5 sets	
Hoops	15	
Geometric Shapes	1 set	
Balls	5	8½" diameter
Ropes	15	8 ft
Jumping Box	1	
Colored Chalk	1 box	
Parachute	1	19½ ft diameter
Movement Music records/tapes	5	
Tape Player/Record Player	1	
Frisbees	5	
Milk Carton Scoops	15	
Ring Toss Set	5 sets	
Beach Balls	5	
Clothespins	1 bag	
Lacing Boards	5	
Beads	5 sets	
Vinyl Shapes	5 sets	
Rhythm Sticks	30 sets	
Peg Boards	5 sets	
Jogger	1	
Foot Launchers	3	

Many of the equipment items used in the program are readily available from your local toy and sporting goods stores and, in some cases, even from the department store chains. Also, many items are available direct from: Front Row Experience, 540 Discovery Bay Blvd., Byron, CA 94514.

! MOVEMENT EDUCATION WORKSHOPS !

For information concerning consulting, in-service training and workshops, contact the author directly.

Write:

Melinda Bossenmeyer
2097 Ontario Ave
Corona, CA 91720

Or call: 714-737-7105

••

! FREE CATALOG !

Send for **Free** catalog of INNOVATIVE CURRICULUM GUIDEBOOKS AND MATER-IALS in Movement Education, Special Education and Perceptual-Motor Development.

Write:

FRONT ROW EXPERIENCE
540 Discovery Bay Blvd.
Byron, CA 94514

Questions? Call 415-634-5710